MY SPRING *Wellness* JOURNAL

Michelle D. Rogers, CPT, CHC, CGFI

michellerogersfitness.com

Michelle Rogers

FITNESS

Michelle Rogers, Inc.
P.O. Box 343, Efland, NC 27243

Find out about online exercise classes, courses, podcast, blog, and online personal training for midlife and older women:
michellerogersfitness.com

Subscribe to free newsletter:
michellerogersfitness.com/newsletter

Connect on Facebook, Instagram, X, Threads, TikTok, YouTube and Pinterest:
@MRhealthyliving

Helpful resources for this journal:
michellerogersfitness.com/journal-resources

Disclaimer

This publication is for informational purposes only. The information presented herein is in no way intended as medical advice or to serve as a substitute for medical counseling. This publication is intended only to supplement, not replace, medical care or advice as part of a healthful lifestyle. As such, the information should be used in conjunction with the guidance and care of your physician. Consult your health care provider before beginning an exercise or nutrition program if you have any pre-existing health conditions or risk factors.

BEING THANKFUL FOR THE BODY YOU HAVE

By Michelle Rogers

The most powerful words in the universe
Are those you whisper to yourself.

What if we stopped obsessing over our flaws
And spoke kinder to ourselves, without pause?

Words that empower us and restore our trust
Giving us strength, not feelings of disgust.

Science says gratitude is good for our health
And writing in a journal daily can help.

We're perfectly imperfect in our own unique way,
So be gentle and appreciate this day by day.

See beauty in yourself and thankfulness will grow,
Let go of judgement and find what you know.

Instead of dwelling on our flaws, let's focus on what's good,
Each time we exercise it should be understood;

Our body is amazing and deserves respect every day,
It works hard to carry us each step of the way.

So when you talk to yourself, make sure it's with care,
Love and gratitude will take you there.

Speak positively and avoid compare.
Cherish you...just as you are...*right here.*

Contents

INTRODUCTION

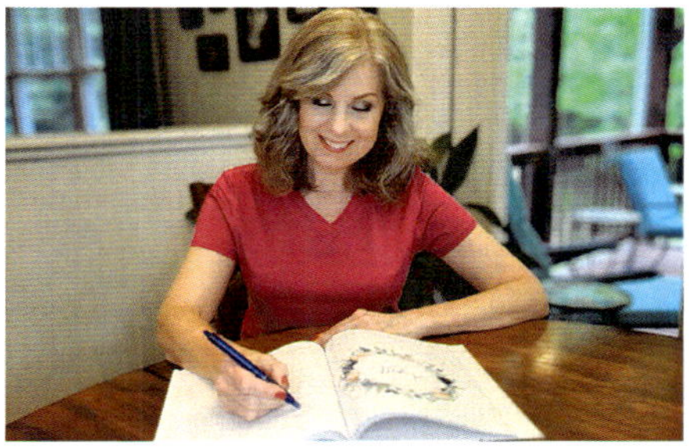

I use my journal daily

Hi, and thank you for purchasing this journal. Let's get to know each other a bit. My name is Michelle Rogers. I am a Certified Personal Trainer, Certified Health Coach, Certified Group Fitness Instructor, Senior Fitness Specialist, and Menopause Health and Fitness Specialist. Most importantly, I'm a proud mother and Mimi to two precious granddaughters.

I was inspired to make a career pivot and become a fitness professional and health coach after taking control of my health and losing a large amount of weight in midlife, and the profound difference that exercise and healthier eating made in every area of my life. After struggling for so long with these issues and finally arriving at success later in life, I was grateful and felt a calling.

Today I'm honored to help other women succeed in their own journeys. I specialize in beginners and moderate-intensity, gentle but effective exercise that helps instead of hurts. And I advocate **the power of small changes for lifestyle transformation that lasts**, rather than restrictive dieting. It's a winning combination that works long-term because it's doable.

I offer online personal training and health coaching exclusively for midlife and older women, and lead online exercise classes and workshops, so if that is something you're interested in please contact me via my website at **michellerogersfitness.com**. I look forward to talking with you!

In addition, I publish a blog and free newsletter where I share tips, news, workouts, recipes and other helpful resources. **Please subscribe to my weekly newsletter** on the website, and follow me on social media at **@MRhealthyliving** so we can stay in touch.

Why I created this journal and what makes it different from others

From the beginning of my weight loss and fitness journey and to this day, logging my daily food and exercise has been **a crucial part** of my strategy to lose and keep off extra pounds, increase my nutrition, stay on track with healthy habits and to help me feel better overall. I also encourage my clients to log.

Over the years I've tried a variety of methods for tracking, including calorie-counting apps and regular notebooks. But none provided exactly what I wanted in a log for myself and my clients. So I created one.

There is power in writing things down on paper. It works like magic. Simply put, when I'm regularly logging my food then I'm losing weight or maintaining. And when I don't log, I'm gaining. For me, there really isn't an in-between.

Menopause hasn't helped any. I've always been the type that puts on weight quickly, but menopause took that to a whole new level (can I get an Amen?!). I've had to be even more intentional with my nutrition and habits. Tracking sleep quality, noticing how something in my diet or exercise affects how I feel, and journaling my thoughts that day are also instrumental in navigating the challenges of menopause and life.

Some people resist the idea of food tracking and call it part of "diet culture." I believe that is a misinformed view, but it's a personal choice—do whatever works for you. From my perspective, keeping a food log is no different than keeping an accurate checkbook: It's data that informs. In the same way that I need to know how much money is in my bank account so that I don't overspend, I want to know the amount of nutrition and activity I should have in my day to keep me healthy, energetic and fit. I want to know how the foods I eat affect me physically and mentally. Journaling has helped me recognize food sensitivities.

As a health coach, I've observed that the main reason people resist logging is because they aren't truly ready to make changes. And that's OK. Despite what many women's magazines and ads would have you believe, there isn't a one-size-fits-all method for diet and exercise and there are no easy quick-fixes that last. If there were, we'd all be perfectly fit.

Rather, it's about finding what works best for **you today**, and that may not be the same thing that worked when you were younger. You don't need to go on a drastic diet or give up your favorite treat; that only leads to yo-yo-ing and defeat. Instead, use this journal to help you see where you can make **small changes** that make sense for you.

Focus on the nutritional quality of what you are eating and drinking, not just the calories. Consume more fresh, whole foods and less that are processed, salty or sugary. You'll be amazed at how much better you feel.

This wellness journal goes further than the traditional calorie-counting we've all done. It gives you a place to track exercise, sleep and your thoughts and feelings that day. The food log lists time of day instead of just meals. **Journaling enables you to make valuable connections between what's going on in your life and what you are eating.**

For example, on days that I'm tired or stressed I'm hungrier and crave potato chips. Research has shown that there is a direct connection between lack of sleep and overeating. But unless I was intentionally thinking about it because of journaling, I may not realize that's what was going on. From journaling, I also realized that when I have sugar it leads to overwhelming cravings for more later that day, often resulting in a binge.

The journal has a full page for each day. Besides giving plenty of space to log, it represents that **each day is literally a new page, a fresh start.** That's an important concept on our wellness journey. And having a designated, pre-dated page to complete each day provides accountability.

Documenting your workouts in the journal's exercise space is also extremely beneficial. It's a great way to note the accomplishment of getting it done, and provides a record you can look back on and see progress. Tracking daily steps? It's a good place for that, too.

Congratulations on choosing to make your health and wellness a priority! As someone who's been there herself and witnessed the powerful impact of exercise and healthier eating in countless others' lives, I can promise you it's a decision you'll be happy you made.

So let's get started.

A FEW WORDS ABOUT CALORIES

Studies have shown that people tend to underestimate how many calories they are consuming, and over-estimate how much they burn with exercise. This can lead to weight gain or stall. Be sure you are tracking ALL of the calories you are consuming, including beverages.

On the other hand, a big mistake some people make is to go too low with calories. Don't think that "the lower the better." That's not sustainable. More importantly, your health and well-being will suffer. Calorie intake should not go below 1,200 calories a day for women and 1,500 for men (Harvard Health). Is that enough food to keep you satisfied to stay on board? For many of us, it may not be necessary to go quite that low in order to lose weight. However, this can vary by individual.

If you exceed the calories per day that your body can use, then the excess is stored as fat. See the chart below for the estimated number of calories your body needs to function. Generally speaking, at that daily calorie amount you'd maintain your weight; over that amount can result in weight gain; and being in a calorie deficit leads to weight loss over time as your body uses stored fat as fuel. It doesn't have to be a drastic deficit for this to work. There's no need to starve yourself.

Estimated Calorie Needs per Day for Females

Age	Sedentary	Moderately Active	Active
31-50	1,800	2,000	2,200
51-60	1,600	1,800	2,200
61 and up	1,600	1,800	2,000

Source: https://www.dietaryguidelines.gov

- Sedentary means a lifestyle that includes only the physical activity of independent living.
- Moderately Active means a lifestyle that includes physical activity equivalent to walking about 1.5 to 3 miles per day at 3 to 4 miles per hour, in addition to the activities of independent living.
- Active means a lifestyle that includes physical activity equivalent to walking more than 3 miles per day at 3 to 4 miles per hour, in addition to the activities of independent living.

Ensure that you are getting proper nutrition, hydration and sleep, which is very important. This journal is a great way to track calories, activity, sleep and macronutrients.

Weight loss is not always just about calories, of course. Hormones, insulin resistance and other health factors can also impact weight and body composition. If you are struggling in this area, see your doctor or a registered dietitian for guidance.

For information about how many calories to eat in order to lose weight, an online calculator, the glycemic index and more, see my journal resources page: **michellerogersfitness.com/journal-resources**.

WHAT ARE MACROS?

The term macros—short for macronutrients—refers to protein, carbohydrates and fats. Macronutrients are the nutrients your body needs in big amounts. Your body breaks down macros for energy to fuel everything you do from breathing to digesting to powering you through your day. But it isn't just about fuel—macros also contain the ingredients your body needs to build and maintain its systems and structures: your muscles, bones, tissues, organs and more. Plus, these large macro groups contain valuable micronutrients, which include vitamins and minerals that your body needs in small amounts—things like iron, calcium and vitamin D. These micronutrients help your body produce the enzymes and hormones to stay healthy.

Protein is essential for muscle growth and helping prevent sarcopenia, the age-related loss in skeletal muscle. Many midlife women don't get enough protein. Your body also needs carbohydrates, especially your brain and muscles. Carbs help power you through exercise. But aim for healthy sources of carbs, rather than sugar. If losing belly fat is a goal, consider limiting the amount of sugar and grains (starchy carbs) in your diet. When going low carb, it may take extra effort to get enough fiber daily, but this is important for good health. That's why this journal's food log includes fiber tracking along with macros.

For more information about calculating macros and determining the right amount for you, see my resources page: **michellerogersfitness.com/journal-resources**.

HOW MUCH SHOULD YOU EXERCISE?

Aging causes loss of bone and muscle mass, but exercise and a healthy diet can help keep you strong and mobile. **Exercise is vital for midlife and older women** to maintain as much muscle and bone mass as we can. Exercise is one of the best ways to slow or prevent problems with the muscles, joints and bones. Remember: "Use it or lose it."

The Physical Activity Guidelines for Americans published by the U.S. Office of Disease Prevention and Health Promotion advises that adults get **at least** 150 to 300 minutes weekly of moderate-intensity aerobic activity, or 75 to 150 minutes weekly of vigorous-intensity aerobic activity, or an equivalent combination of both, plus muscle-strengthening activities on at least two days a week.

150 minutes weekly equals 30 minutes, five days a week. If you participate in my online exercise classes, you'll meet the recommended weekly amount of moderate-intensity cardio and strength work. What I recommend for a client will depend on her current level of fitness, her goals and any health conditions. For a beginner exercising on their own, I generally recommend starting with a small amount—15-30 minutes a day of moderate intensity—and working up to more over time.

A half-hour workout is just 2% of your day. But know that **any amount of exercise you do, no matter how small, is better than nothing and will benefit you.** The main thing is to focus on making exercise a daily habit. Set a scheduled time to exercise in your calendar, and give it the priority of an important meeting.

That's one of the advantages of taking professionally-led classes or working with a certified personal trainer. It's an appointment to exercise, the exercises are programmed for you, and it takes the guesswork out of working out. Learn more about my online exercise classes and online personal training services for women over 50 at **michellerogersfitness.com**.

HOW TO USE THIS JOURNAL

- Keep your journal in a visible, convenient place so that you are reminded to log.
- Log your food, beverages and exercise as it happens, so that you are remembering it clearly. Or, you can use the log as a meal planner and then check things off.
- What you log is up to you. You don't have to count calories or figure out the macros, if you don't want to.
- If you're just getting started or are new to tracking, I advise logging your foods and beverages without figuring the calories or macros, at least the first week. The idea is to simply become aware of what your daily intake looks like.
- You can use a calorie counting app or website to determine the calories and macronutrients. If it's a packaged food, use the nutrition facts label. Be accurate about the portion size so that you don't underestimate.
- This journal is adaptable to your needs. For example, if you're following Weight Watchers, you could log points instead of calories in that space. Or perhaps, you only want to log your exercise and thoughts.
- Remember that it isn't about being perfect. If you get off track and forget to log, or have an overindulgence, just start back up the next day. It's not all or nothing!

WHAT IS YOUR "WHY"?

Start with your purpose. What is your "why"? Write it below. Refer to it regularly as a reminder of your true motivation.

Why do you want to get in shape? To feel less stiff and sore? To have more energy? To prevent or reverse type-2 diabetes? To be able to get down on the floor to play with kids? To have more confidence?

This should be about more than solely achieving a certain size or weight. Envision yourself having reached your goal. How would your life be different?

Measurements Log

	Start date: ______	April	May	June	Total inches lost
Neck (largest part)					
Chest (across bust)					
Waist (smallest part)					
Belly (below belly button)					
Hips (largest part)					
Left thigh (largest part)					
Right thigh					
Upper arm: Left bicep *					
Right bicep *					
Lower arm: Left forearm *					
Right forearm *					
Left calf * (largest part)					
Right calf *					

**Optional*

- **When to take measurements and weight:** First thing in the morning, after using the bathroom, with no clothes on, and before having any food or drink. Make sure the scale is on a flat surface, not carpet.
- If weight loss is a goal, I suggest tracking weight weekly (not daily) and measurements monthly. It is normal for weight to fluctuate from day to day due to water retention.
- On the other hand, if using a scale doesn't feel right for you (for some it can be triggering and lead to self-sabotage), *then don't weigh yourself at all.* That's right—ditch the scale!
- Be patient. Body transformation takes time and persistence. Accept that it may take longer than you might like, even if you are doing all the right things. This is especially true for midlife and older women.
- Focus primarily on developing the habits of exercise and healthier eating, rather than just on weight and body size. Make it about a lifestyle you can sustain long term, rather than going on a diet.
- Plateaus and setbacks are a normal part of the process. Don't give up.

Weight Log

Date	Weight	Total pounds lost

5 ways to measure progress that have nothing to do with pounds:

1. **Body composition**. Often you'll see changes in measurements first, more so than pounds (especially with exercise). If you have a smart scale, you can easily track body fat percentage, too. Or, just go by how your clothes feel.
2. **Well-being and stamina.** Is your mood, stress level or quality of sleep improving? Are you feeling stronger, more energetic, more flexible or less stiff and sore?
3. **Fitness level.** Are you able to do activities of daily living better than before, like yard work? Getting more steps in each day? Or able to lift more weight or do more reps?
4. **Health.** With healthier eating and exercise you should see improvements in your blood pressure, blood sugar, cholesterol and other levels, over time.
5. **Habits.** If you've succeeded in incorporating a healthier habit into your life, such as a daily walk, or less fast food, this is major progress! Our habits form the foundation of all success. Keep up the great work.

April

MY GOALS FOR APRIL

MY EXERCISE PLAN FOR APRIL

MY HEALTHY EATING PLAN FOR APRIL

Success tip: Keep your plan simple and doable! Consider focusing on just ONE thing in these areas, rather than making a long list.

APRIL 1

Today's exercise

How I slept

Time	Food/Beverage	Calories	Protein (grams)	Carbs (grams)	Fat (grams)	Fiber (grams)
	TOTAL					

Thoughts and Feelings

APRIL 2

Today's exercise

How I slept

Time	Food/Beverage	Calories	Protein (grams)	Carbs (grams)	Fat (grams)	Fiber (grams)
	TOTAL					

Thoughts and Feelings

APRIL 3

Today's exercise

How I slept

Time	Food/Beverage	Calories	Protein (grams)	Carbs (grams)	Fat (grams)	Fiber (grams)
	TOTAL					

Thoughts and Feelings

APRIL 4

Today's exercise

How I slept

Time	Food/Beverage	Calories	Protein (grams)	Carbs (grams)	Fat (grams)	Fiber (grams)
	TOTAL					

Thoughts and Feelings

APRIL 5

Today's exercise

How I slept

Time	Food/Beverage	Calories	Protein (grams)	Carbs (grams)	Fat (grams)	Fiber (grams)
	TOTAL					

Thoughts and Feelings

APRIL 6

Today's exercise

How I slept

Time	Food/Beverage	Calories	Protein (grams)	Carbs (grams)	Fat (grams)	Fiber (grams)
	TOTAL					

Thoughts and Feelings

APRIL 7

Today's exercise

How I slept

Time	Food/Beverage	Calories	Protein (grams)	Carbs (grams)	Fat (grams)	Fiber (grams)
	TOTAL					

Thoughts and Feelings

APRIL 8

Today's exercise

How I slept

Time	Food/Beverage	Calories	Protein (grams)	Carbs (grams)	Fat (grams)	Fiber (grams)
	TOTAL					

Thoughts and Feelings

APRIL 9

Today's exercise

How I slept

Time	Food/Beverage	Calories	Protein (grams)	Carbs (grams)	Fat (grams)	Fiber (grams)
	TOTAL					

Thoughts and Feelings

APRIL 10

Today's exercise

How I slept

Time	Food/Beverage	Calories	Protein (grams)	Carbs (grams)	Fat (grams)	Fiber (grams)
	TOTAL					

Thoughts and Feelings

APRIL 11

Today's exercise

How I slept

Time	Food/Beverage	Calories	Protein (grams)	Carbs (grams)	Fat (grams)	Fiber (grams)
	TOTAL					

Thoughts and Feelings

APRIL 12

Today's exercise

How I slept

Time	Food/Beverage	Calories	Protein (grams)	Carbs (grams)	Fat (grams)	Fiber (grams)
	TOTAL					

Thoughts and Feelings

APRIL 13

Today's exercise

How I slept

Time	Food/Beverage	Calories	Protein (grams)	Carbs (grams)	Fat (grams)	Fiber (grams)
	TOTAL					

Thoughts and Feelings

APRIL 14

Today's exercise

How I slept

Time	Food/Beverage	Calories	Protein (grams)	Carbs (grams)	Fat (grams)	Fiber (grams)
	TOTAL					

Thoughts and Feelings

APRIL 15

Today's exercise

How I slept

Time	Food/Beverage	Calories	Protein (grams)	Carbs (grams)	Fat (grams)	Fiber (grams)
	TOTAL					

Thoughts and Feelings

APRIL 16

Today's exercise

How I slept

Time	Food/Beverage	Calories	Protein (grams)	Carbs (grams)	Fat (grams)	Fiber (grams)
	TOTAL					

Thoughts and Feelings

APRIL 17

Today's exercise

How I slept

Time	Food/Beverage	Calories	Protein (grams)	Carbs (grams)	Fat (grams)	Fiber (grams)
	TOTAL					

Thoughts and Feelings

Today's exercise

How I slept

Time	Food/Beverage	Calories	Protein (grams)	Carbs (grams)	Fat (grams)	Fiber (grams)
	TOTAL					

Thoughts and Feelings

APRIL 19

Today's exercise

How I slept

Time	Food/Beverage	Calories	Protein (grams)	Carbs (grams)	Fat (grams)	Fiber (grams)
	TOTAL					

Thoughts and Feelings

Today's exercise

How I slept

Time	Food/Beverage	Calories	Protein (grams)	Carbs (grams)	Fat (grams)	Fiber (grams)
	TOTAL					

Thoughts and Feelings

APRIL 21

Today's exercise

How I slept

Time	Food/Beverage	Calories	Protein (grams)	Carbs (grams)	Fat (grams)	Fiber (grams)
	TOTAL					

Thoughts and Feelings

APRIL 22

Today's exercise

How I slept

Time	Food/Beverage	Calories	Protein (grams)	Carbs (grams)	Fat (grams)	Fiber (grams)
	TOTAL					

Thoughts and Feelings

APRIL 23

Today's exercise

How I slept

Time	Food/Beverage	Calories	Protein (grams)	Carbs (grams)	Fat (grams)	Fiber (grams)
	TOTAL					

Thoughts and Feelings

APRIL 24

Today's exercise

How I slept

Time	Food/Beverage	Calories	Protein (grams)	Carbs (grams)	Fat (grams)	Fiber (grams)
	TOTAL					

Thoughts and Feelings

APRIL 25

Today's exercise

How I slept

Time	Food/Beverage	Calories	Protein (grams)	Carbs (grams)	Fat (grams)	Fiber (grams)
	TOTAL					

Thoughts and Feelings

APRIL 26

Today's exercise

How I slept

Time	Food/Beverage	Calories	Protein (grams)	Carbs (grams)	Fat (grams)	Fiber (grams)
	TOTAL					

Thoughts and Feelings

APRIL 27

Today's exercise

How I slept

Time	Food/Beverage	Calories	Protein (grams)	Carbs (grams)	Fat (grams)	Fiber (grams)
	TOTAL					

Thoughts and Feelings

APRIL 28

Today's exercise

How I slept

Time	Food/Beverage	Calories	Protein (grams)	Carbs (grams)	Fat (grams)	Fiber (grams)
	TOTAL					

Thoughts and Feelings

APRIL 29

Today's exercise

How I slept

Time	Food/Beverage	Calories	Protein (grams)	Carbs (grams)	Fat (grams)	Fiber (grams)
	TOTAL					

Thoughts and Feelings

APRIL 30

Today's exercise

How I slept

Time	Food/Beverage	Calories	Protein (grams)	Carbs (grams)	Fat (grams)	Fiber (grams)
	TOTAL					

Thoughts and Feelings

April
REVIEW

WHAT I DID WELL THIS MONTH

SOMETHING I WOULD LIKE TO IMPROVE AND KEEP WORKING ON

WHAT DIFFERENCES AM I SEEING OR FEELING IN MY BODY AND MIND SINCE I STARTED?

Help is here!

You don't need to go it alone or struggle in your journey.
Let's work together, to help you succeed!

Online exercise classes for midlife and older adults and beginners

Online courses

Live online one-on-one personal training and wellness coaching for midlife and older women, specializing in gentle fitness

Learn more at **michellerogersfitness.com**

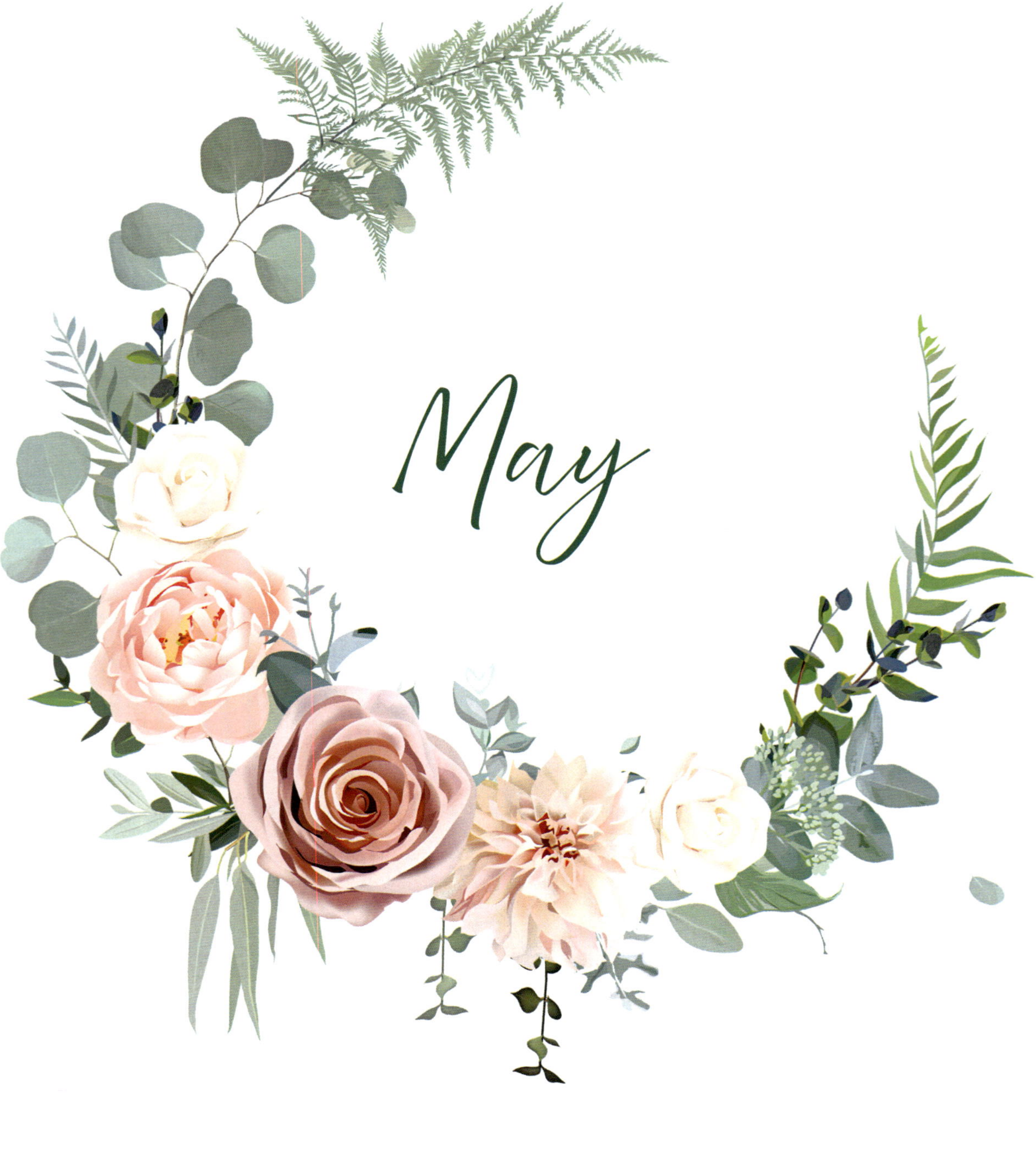

May

MY GOALS FOR MAY

MY EXERCISE PLAN FOR MAY

MY HEALTHY EATING PLAN FOR MAY

Success tip: Keep your plan simple and doable! Consider focusing on just ONE thing in these areas, rather than making a long list.

MAY 1

Today's exercise

How I slept

Time	Food/Beverage	Calories	Protein (grams)	Carbs (grams)	Fat (grams)	Fiber (grams)
	TOTAL					

Thoughts and Feelings

MAY 2

Today's exercise

How I slept

Time	Food/Beverage	Calories	Protein (grams)	Carbs (grams)	Fat (grams)	Fiber (grams)
	TOTAL					

Thoughts and Feelings

MAY 3

Today's exercise

How I slept

Time	Food/Beverage	Calories	Protein (grams)	Carbs (grams)	Fat (grams)	Fiber (grams)
	TOTAL					

Thoughts and Feelings

MAY 4

Today's exercise

How I slept

Time	Food/Beverage	Calories	Protein (grams)	Carbs (grams)	Fat (grams)	Fiber (grams)
	TOTAL					

Thoughts and Feelings

MAY 5

Today's exercise

How I slept

Time	Food/Beverage	Calories	Protein (grams)	Carbs (grams)	Fat (grams)	Fiber (grams)
	TOTAL					

Thoughts and Feelings

MAY 6

Today's exercise

How I slept

Time	Food/Beverage	Calories	Protein (grams)	Carbs (grams)	Fat (grams)	Fiber (grams)
	TOTAL					

Thoughts and Feelings

MAY 7

Today's exercise

How I slept

Time	Food/Beverage	Calories	Protein (grams)	Carbs (grams)	Fat (grams)	Fiber (grams)
	TOTAL					

Thoughts and Feelings

MAY 8

Today's exercise

How I slept

Time	Food/Beverage	Calories	Protein (grams)	Carbs (grams)	Fat (grams)	Fiber (grams)
	TOTAL					

Thoughts and Feelings

MAY 9

Today's exercise

How I slept

Time	Food/Beverage	Calories	Protein (grams)	Carbs (grams)	Fat (grams)	Fiber (grams)
	TOTAL					

Thoughts and Feelings

MAY 10

Today's exercise

How I slept

Time	Food/Beverage	Calories	Protein (grams)	Carbs (grams)	Fat (grams)	Fiber (grams)
	TOTAL					

Thoughts and Feelings

MAY 11

Today's exercise

How I slept

Time	Food/Beverage	Calories	Protein (grams)	Carbs (grams)	Fat (grams)	Fiber (grams)
	TOTAL					

Thoughts and Feelings

MAY 12

Today's exercise

How I slept

Time	Food/Beverage	Calories	Protein (grams)	Carbs (grams)	Fat (grams)	Fiber (grams)
	TOTAL					

Thoughts and Feelings

MAY 13

Today's exercise

How I slept

Time	Food/Beverage	Calories	Protein (grams)	Carbs (grams)	Fat (grams)	Fiber (grams)
	TOTAL					

Thoughts and Feelings

MAY 14

Today's exercise

How I slept

Time	Food/Beverage	Calories	Protein (grams)	Carbs (grams)	Fat (grams)	Fiber (grams)
	TOTAL					

Thoughts and Feelings

MAY 15

Today's exercise

How I slept

Time	Food/Beverage	Calories	Protein (grams)	Carbs (grams)	Fat (grams)	Fiber (grams)
	TOTAL					

Thoughts and Feelings

MAY 16

Today's exercise

How I slept

Time	Food/Beverage	Calories	Protein (grams)	Carbs (grams)	Fat (grams)	Fiber (grams)
	TOTAL					

Thoughts and Feelings

Today's exercise

How I slept

Time	Food/Beverage	Calories	Protein (grams)	Carbs (grams)	Fat (grams)	Fiber (grams)
	TOTAL					

Thoughts and Feelings

MAY 18

Today's exercise

How I slept

Time	Food/Beverage	Calories	Protein (grams)	Carbs (grams)	Fat (grams)	Fiber (grams)
	TOTAL					

Thoughts and Feelings

MAY 19

Today's exercise

How I slept

Time	Food/Beverage	Calories	Protein (grams)	Carbs (grams)	Fat (grams)	Fiber (grams)
	TOTAL					

Thoughts and Feelings

MAY 20

Today's exercise

How I slept

Time	Food/Beverage	Calories	Protein (grams)	Carbs (grams)	Fat (grams)	Fiber (grams)
	TOTAL					

Thoughts and Feelings

MAY 21

Today's exercise

How I slept

Time	Food/Beverage	Calories	Protein (grams)	Carbs (grams)	Fat (grams)	Fiber (grams)
	TOTAL					

Thoughts and Feelings

MAY 22

Today's exercise

How I slept

Time	Food/Beverage	Calories	Protein (grams)	Carbs (grams)	Fat (grams)	Fiber (grams)
	TOTAL					

Thoughts and Feelings

MAY 23

Today's exercise

How I slept

Time	Food/Beverage	Calories	Protein (grams)	Carbs (grams)	Fat (grams)	Fiber (grams)
	TOTAL					

Thoughts and Feelings

MAY 24

Today's exercise

How I slept

Time	Food/Beverage	Calories	Protein (grams)	Carbs (grams)	Fat (grams)	Fiber (grams)
	TOTAL					

Thoughts and Feelings

MAY 25

Today's exercise

How I slept

Time	Food/Beverage	Calories	Protein (grams)	Carbs (grams)	Fat (grams)	Fiber (grams)
	TOTAL					

Thoughts and Feelings

MAY 26

Today's exercise

How I slept

Time	Food/Beverage	Calories	Protein (grams)	Carbs (grams)	Fat (grams)	Fiber (grams)
	TOTAL					

Thoughts and Feelings

MAY 27

Today's exercise

How I slept

Time	Food/Beverage	Calories	Protein (grams)	Carbs (grams)	Fat (grams)	Fiber (grams)
	TOTAL					

Thoughts and Feelings

MAY 28

Today's exercise

How I slept

Time	Food/Beverage	Calories	Protein (grams)	Carbs (grams)	Fat (grams)	Fiber (grams)
	TOTAL					

Thoughts and Feelings

MAY 29

Today's exercise

How I slept

Time	Food/Beverage	Calories	Protein (grams)	Carbs (grams)	Fat (grams)	Fiber (grams)
	TOTAL					

Thoughts and Feelings

MAY 30

Today's exercise

How I slept

Time	Food/Beverage	Calories	Protein (grams)	Carbs (grams)	Fat (grams)	Fiber (grams)
	TOTAL					

Thoughts and Feelings

Today's exercise

How I slept

Time	Food/Beverage	Calories	Protein (grams)	Carbs (grams)	Fat (grams)	Fiber (grams)
	TOTAL					

Thoughts and Feelings

May
REVIEW

WHAT I DID WELL THIS MONTH

SOMETHING I WOULD LIKE TO IMPROVE AND KEEP WORKING ON

WHAT DIFFERENCES AM I SEEING OR FEELING IN MY BODY AND MIND SINCE I STARTED?

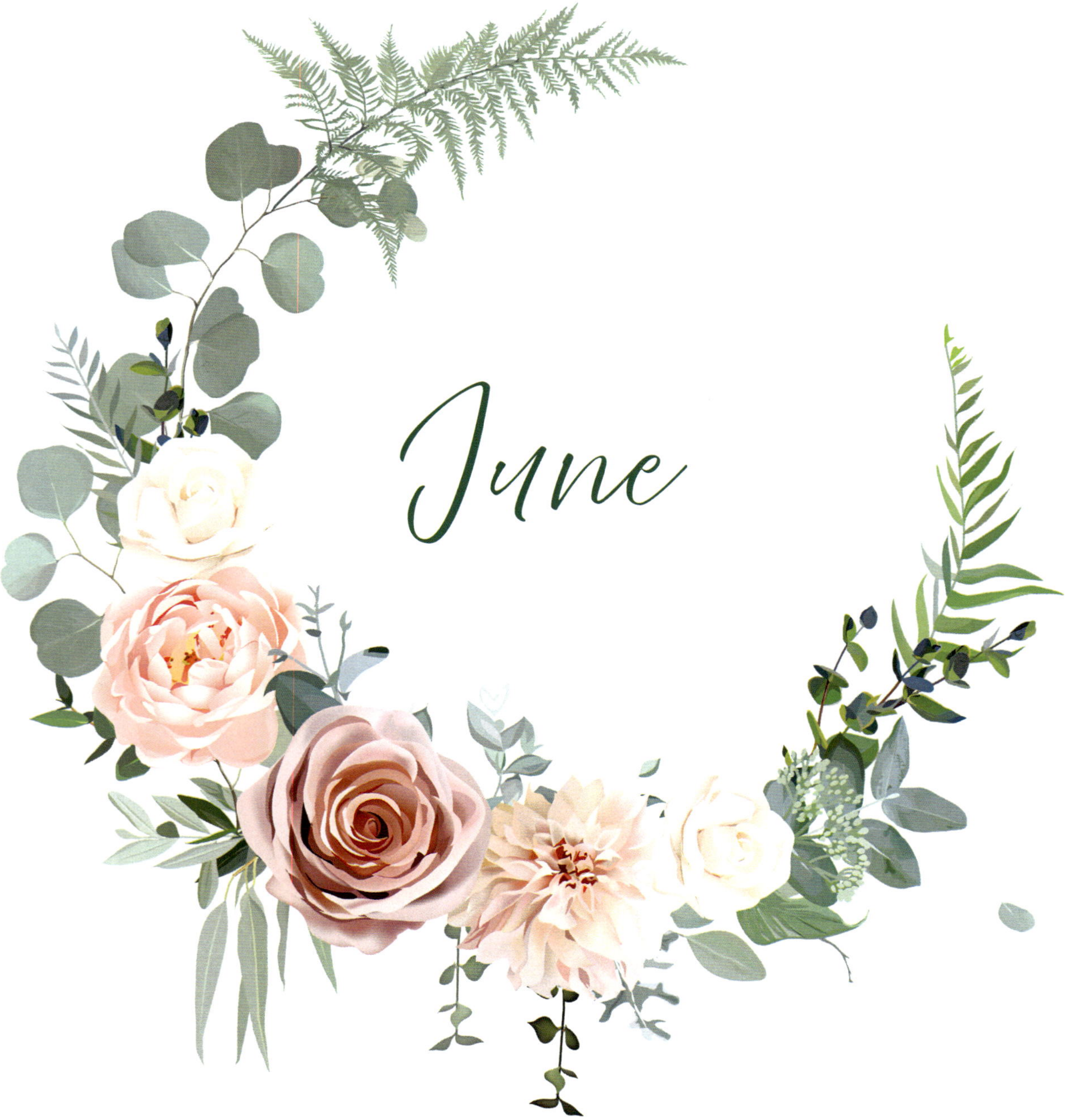

June

MY GOALS FOR JUNE

MY EXERCISE PLAN FOR JUNE

MY HEALTHY EATING PLAN FOR JUNE

Success tip: Keep your plan simple and doable! Consider focusing on just ONE thing in these areas, rather than making a long list.

TIME TO ORDER YOUR SUMMER WELLNESS JOURNAL

at michellerogersfitness.com

Today's exercise

How I slept

Time	Food/Beverage	Calories	Protein (grams)	Carbs (grams)	Fat (grams)	Fiber (grams)
	TOTAL					

Thoughts and Feelings

Today's exercise

How I slept

Time	Food/Beverage	Calories	Protein (grams)	Carbs (grams)	Fat (grams)	Fiber (grams)
	TOTAL					

Thoughts and Feelings

JUNE 3

Today's exercise

How I slept

Time	Food/Beverage	Calories	Protein (grams)	Carbs (grams)	Fat (grams)	Fiber (grams)
	TOTAL					

Thoughts and Feelings

JUNE 4

Today's exercise

How I slept

Time	Food/Beverage	Calories	Protein (grams)	Carbs (grams)	Fat (grams)	Fiber (grams)
	TOTAL					

Thoughts and Feelings

Today's exercise

How I slept

Time	Food/Beverage	Calories	Protein (grams)	Carbs (grams)	Fat (grams)	Fiber (grams)
	TOTAL					

Thoughts and Feelings

JUNE 6

Today's exercise

How I slept

Time	Food/Beverage	Calories	Protein (grams)	Carbs (grams)	Fat (grams)	Fiber (grams)
	TOTAL					

Thoughts and Feelings

JUNE 7

Today's exercise

How I slept

Time	Food/Beverage	Calories	Protein (grams)	Carbs (grams)	Fat (grams)	Fiber (grams)
	TOTAL					

Thoughts and Feelings

JUNE 8

Today's exercise

How I slept

Time	Food/Beverage	Calories	Protein (grams)	Carbs (grams)	Fat (grams)	Fiber (grams)
	TOTAL					

Thoughts and Feelings

JUNE 9

Today's exercise

How I slept

Time	Food/Beverage	Calories	Protein (grams)	Carbs (grams)	Fat (grams)	Fiber (grams)
	TOTAL					

Thoughts and Feelings

JUNE 10

Today's exercise

How I slept

Time	Food/Beverage	Calories	Protein (grams)	Carbs (grams)	Fat (grams)	Fiber (grams)
	TOTAL					

Thoughts and Feelings

JUNE 11

Today's exercise

How I slept

Time	Food/Beverage	Calories	Protein (grams)	Carbs (grams)	Fat (grams)	Fiber (grams)
	TOTAL					

Thoughts and Feelings

JUNE 12

Today's exercise

How I slept

Time	Food/Beverage	Calories	Protein (grams)	Carbs (grams)	Fat (grams)	Fiber (grams)
	TOTAL					

Thoughts and Feelings

JUNE 13

Today's exercise

How I slept

Time	Food/Beverage	Calories	Protein (grams)	Carbs (grams)	Fat (grams)	Fiber (grams)
	TOTAL					

Thoughts and Feelings

JUNE 14

Today's exercise

How I slept

Time	Food/Beverage	Calories	Protein (grams)	Carbs (grams)	Fat (grams)	Fiber (grams)
	TOTAL					

Thoughts and Feelings

JUNE 15

Today's exercise

How I slept

Time	Food/Beverage	Calories	Protein (grams)	Carbs (grams)	Fat (grams)	Fiber (grams)
	TOTAL					

Thoughts and Feelings

JUNE 16

Today's exercise

How I slept

Time	Food/Beverage	Calories	Protein (grams)	Carbs (grams)	Fat (grams)	Fiber (grams)
	TOTAL					

Thoughts and Feelings

JUNE 17

Today's exercise

How I slept

Time	Food/Beverage	Calories	Protein (grams)	Carbs (grams)	Fat (grams)	Fiber (grams)
	TOTAL					

Thoughts and Feelings

JUNE 18

Today's exercise

How I slept

Time	Food/Beverage	Calories	Protein (grams)	Carbs (grams)	Fat (grams)	Fiber (grams)
	TOTAL					

Thoughts and Feelings

JUNE 19

Today's exercise

How I slept

Time	Food/Beverage	Calories	Protein (grams)	Carbs (grams)	Fat (grams)	Fiber (grams)
	TOTAL					

Thoughts and Feelings

JUNE 20

Today's exercise

How I slept

Time	Food/Beverage	Calories	Protein (grams)	Carbs (grams)	Fat (grams)	Fiber (grams)
	TOTAL					

Thoughts and Feelings

JUNE 21

Today's exercise

How I slept

Time	Food/Beverage	Calories	Protein (grams)	Carbs (grams)	Fat (grams)	Fiber (grams)
	TOTAL					

Thoughts and Feelings

Today's exercise

How I slept

Time	Food/Beverage	Calories	Protein (grams)	Carbs (grams)	Fat (grams)	Fiber (grams)
	TOTAL					

Thoughts and Feelings

JUNE 23

Today's exercise

How I slept

Time	Food/Beverage	Calories	Protein (grams)	Carbs (grams)	Fat (grams)	Fiber (grams)
	TOTAL					

Thoughts and Feelings

JUNE 24

Today's exercise

How I slept

Time	Food/Beverage	Calories	Protein (grams)	Carbs (grams)	Fat (grams)	Fiber (grams)
	TOTAL					

Thoughts and Feelings

JUNE 25

Today's exercise

How I slept

Time	Food/Beverage	Calories	Protein (grams)	Carbs (grams)	Fat (grams)	Fiber (grams)
	TOTAL					

Thoughts and Feelings

JUNE 26

Today's exercise

How I slept

Time	Food/Beverage	Calories	Protein (grams)	Carbs (grams)	Fat (grams)	Fiber (grams)
	TOTAL					

Thoughts and Feelings

JUNE 27

Today's exercise

How I slept

Time	Food/Beverage	Calories	Protein (grams)	Carbs (grams)	Fat (grams)	Fiber (grams)
	TOTAL					

Thoughts and Feelings

JUNE 28

Today's exercise

How I slept

Time	Food/Beverage	Calories	Protein (grams)	Carbs (grams)	Fat (grams)	Fiber (grams)
	TOTAL					

Thoughts and Feelings

JUNE 29

Today's exercise

How I slept

Time	Food/Beverage	Calories	Protein (grams)	Carbs (grams)	Fat (grams)	Fiber (grams)
	TOTAL					

Thoughts and Feelings

JUNE 30

Today's exercise

How I slept

Time	Food/Beverage	Calories	Protein (grams)	Carbs (grams)	Fat (grams)	Fiber (grams)
	TOTAL					

Thoughts and Feelings

June

REVIEW

WHAT I DID WELL THIS MONTH

SOMETHING I WOULD LIKE TO IMPROVE AND KEEP WORKING ON

WHAT DIFFERENCES AM I SEEING OR FEELING IN MY BODY AND MIND SINCE I STARTED?

CONGRATULATIONS!
KEEP UP THE
GREAT WORK!

KEEP LOGGING.
BE PATIENT.
DON'T GIVE UP!

ORDER YOUR
SUMMER, FALL AND WINTER
WELLNESS JOURNALS

at michellerogersfitness.com

Help is here!

You don't need to go it alone or struggle in your journey.
Let's work together, to help you succeed!
I offer:

Online exercise classes for midlife and older adults and beginners

Online courses

Live online one-on-one personal training and health coaching for midlife and older women, specializing in beginners

Learn more at **michellerogersfitness.com**

Notes

Made in United States
North Haven, CT
05 November 2026

21765022R00066